ৡ Amoxicillin ৢ

The Excellent Guide to Treat STDs like Gonorrhea, Syphilis; Pneumonia, Dental Abscess, **Stomach Ulcer, Skin, Nose, Ear Infections etc., by Using Amoxicillin & be Side Effect-Free**

Dr. Lovel Martins

Table of Contents

3

❧ Introduction ❧

Amoxicillin was originated in the early 1970s in the United Kingdom. It is a broad spectrum antibacterial that helps in the treatment of several diseases.

Amoxicillin is very effective against both gram positive and gram negative micro-organisms in humans and animals: and it also possesses higher efficiency compared to penicillin.

Infections were listed as the primary cause of infant death and the primary source of disease burden globally by the World Health Organization (WHO) in 2005. The most common infectious cause of mortality in people of all ages is acute respiratory infections.

One of the penicillin antibiotic subtypes used to combat a variety of diseases and inflammations is amoxicillin. Some disease-causing organisms may be the source of these illnesses.

Numerous infections and inflammations are brought on by various bacteria, fungi, viruses, etc., according to research. It is said that humans are vulnerable to these disease-causing microbes through a variety of media, including food, drink, and the air.

The existence of these numerous disease-causing organisms ended up causing countless types of infections in the body, including burns, wounds, boils, impetigo infections, erysipelas, carbuncles, acne, and Sexually Transmitted Diseases (STDs) like Gonorrhea, Chlamydia, and Syphilis; Respiratory diseases like Pneumonia, Whooping Cough, Tuberculosis, Scarlet Fever, and Legionnaires Disease.

Leprosy, tetanus, meningitis, and botulism are diseases of the nervous system, as are typhoid fever, diphtheria, and plague, which affect the body's whole systemic circulation.

To stop them from spreading from an infected person to an uninfected person, they all need competent clinical care. Patients will benefit more from Amoxicillin treatment if their infections are still in the early stages.

It is advised to keep Amoxicillin on hand as first aid for combating any infectious or contagious sickness that occurs through water, food, air, or soil in the environment. As a result, those with impaired immune systems or immunological deficiencies may catch the infection right away.

Apart from using Amoxicillin to combat bacterial infections, it could also be used as prophylaxis against endocarditis caused by bacterial and tooth care.

Amoxicillin is also compared with other antibiotics such as Azithromycin, Clarithromycin, Ampicillin, Cefuroxime and Doxycycline. All these antibiotics are very powerful and are capable to fight bacterial infections.

In this book, I am going to expose you to the basis of Amoxicillin, its working mechanisms, its medical benefits, all the infections that could be treated with this pill, its side effects and some interactions that might occur with the use of this pill concomitantly with other medication.

Also, you are expected to consult your Doctor before you take any medication including Amoxicillin. Your Doctor will give you the appropriate advice that you need.

Chapter One

Understanding Amoxicillin

Amoxicillin is a penicillin-class antibiotic, along with ampicillin, piperacillin, and others. This medicine is employed to treat a wide range of bacterial disorders.

Antibiotics with the same healing process are grouped together under the name Penicillin products. They do not immediately destroy bacteria. They prevent or make it more difficult for the bacteria cells to grow and reproduce in the surrounding wall that directs them.

These walls serve as a barrier between the bacterium cell and its immediate surroundings and are crucial for tying each cell together into a cord. It is challenging for the bacteria cells to live outside of the cell wall.

By preventing the growth of bacteria that cause illnesses from multiplying or reproducing, amoxicillin prevents the occurrence of bacterial infections. Amoxicillin medication breaks down the infecting bacteria's protective cell wall, exposing the nucleolus, a concentrated organelle inside the cell that contains the genetic material chromatin, ribonucleic acid (RNA), and proteins.

When the life-determinant nucleolus of bacteria is exposed, the contagious germs in the victim's body are killed or destroyed.

Amoxicillin may be used to treat duodenal ulcers brought on by Helicobacter pylori. Before it may treat a duodenal ulcer, this medicine must be administered concurrently with other medicines (antibiotics), such as clarithromycin.

Another over-the-counter antibiotic used to treat illnesses brought on by several types of bacteria is amoxicillin. It could be utilized in a combined treatment. This suggests that, if necessary, you might combine amoxicillin with other drugs.

Children often receive amoxicillin treatment for chest and ear infections. This may come in liquid or injectable form.

Amoxicillin oral pills are available as chewable, immediate-release, and extended-release tablets. There are no brand-name medications in chewable or extended-release forms.

The History of Amoxicillin Creation

The fundamental nucleus of Penicillins is a lactam ring, and in neutral or basic conditions, this ring can be opened, producing an inert medication. Lactamase, a bacterial enzyme that may break down Penicillin antibiotics, also interacts with the ring.

As a result, chemical structures must be introduced to penicillin antibiotics to boost their acid consistency and - lactamase resistance.

By making the amide oxygen less nucleophilic, as in amoxicillin, the addition of an electron withdrawing group to the amide group in the sixth position might boost the acid stability of the compound. This makes sure that the carbonyl group of the lactam ring won't be attacked by the amide oxygen and opened.

Penicillin G and penicillin V were the only two antibiotics in the 1950s' whole "lactam" family that had a wide range of action.

There was a great deal of interest in creating novel penicillin by changing the molecule's side chain. The side chain donors might be added to the fermentation broth as one technique. However, the number and variety of chemicals that could be created in this manner were constrained.

The Chemical Properties of Amoxicillin

Amoxicillin comes in powder form that is white or almost white, has a faint sulfurous odor, and is compatible with buffers made of citrate, phosphate, and borate.

While amoxicillin trihydrate hardly dissolved in water, barely soluble in ethanol, and essentially insoluble in fatty oils, amoxicillin sodium is extremely soluble in water, slightly soluble in anhydrous ethanol, and very marginally soluble in acetone. In diluted acid and alkali hydroxide solutions, it dissolves.

Amoxicillin trihydrate and sodium breakdown were seen to exhibit two-step breakdown in both sealed and open containers at varied temperatures.

Both the amoxicillin trihydrate and the amoxicillin sodium exhibited first order breakdown under regulated humidity conditions.

According to published research, amoxicillin was shown to follow a first order or pseudo-first order degradation rate at stable pH levels, with a minimum rate at around pH 6.

Amoxicillin breakdown was catalyzed by citrate and phosphate buffers, with phosphate causing a 10-fold increase in rate. It has been shown that increasing ionic strength has a beneficial impact on the rate of degradation in alkali and a negative impact on acid.

Amoxicillin had non-first order breakdown rates at higher concentrations, which is indicative of a dimerization process.

At pH 9, amoxicillin dimerizes more quickly than other aminopenicillins. Amoxicillin's degradation at greater concentrations was accelerated by the presence of carbs and alcohols.

Amoxicillin demonstrated pH-dependent stability, with stability rising as pH below 6. Amoxicillin appeared to be degraded in buffered solutions by an acid-base reaction.

Chapter Two

What is Amoxicillin's Mechanism of Action?

A potent antibiotic, amoxicillin destroys germs. It directly kill germs, it prevents them from proliferating and developing inside the body, which prevents them from building a cell wall to protect them.

The bacterial cell wall is rendered ineffective by the "mucopeptides" in the cell wall, which then causes the cell wall to be destroyed.

The walls are essential to keep bacteria safe from their immediate surroundings and to keep the entire bacterial cell intact. A cell wall is essential for the survival of bacteria cells.

Amoxicillin inhibits penicillin-binding protein as well as other higher molecular weight penicillin binding proteins by competitive inhibition.

Penicillin-binding proteins are in charge of the transpeptidase and glycosyltransferase activities that cause D-alanine and D-aspartic acid to cross-link in bacterial cell walls.

Bactericidal effect results from bacteria's inability to construct and repair their cell walls and an upregulation of autolytic enzymes caused by the absence of penicillin binding proteins.

Selective Toxicity of Amoxicillin and other Antimicrobial Drugs

Medically useful antimicrobial drugs exhibit selective toxicity, causing greater harm to microorganisms than to the human host.

They do this by interfering with essential biological structures or biochemical processes that are common in microorganisms but not in human cells.

While the ideal antimicrobial drug is non-toxic to humans, most can be harmful at high concentration. In other words, selective toxicity is a relative term. The toxicity of a given drug is expressed as the therapeutic index, which is the lowest dose toxic to the patient divided by the dose typically used for therapy.

Antimicrobial drugs that have a high therapeutic index are less toxic to the patient, often because the drug acts against a vital biochemical process of bacteria that does not exist in human cells.

For example, penicillin, which interferes with bacteria cell wall synthesis, has a very high therapeutic index. When an antimicrobial drug that has a low therapeutic index is administered, the concentration in the patient's blood must be carefully monitored to ensure it does not reach a toxic level.

Drugs that are too toxic for systemic use can sometimes be used for topical applications, such as first-aid antibiotic skin ointments. However, Amoxicillin is not a toxic antibiotic, hence; it can be administered for internal use.

The Antimicrobial Action of Amoxicillin

Antimicrobial drugs can either kill an organism or inhibit their growth. Those that inhibit growth are called bacteriostatic. These drugs depend on the normal host defenses to kill or eliminate the pathogen after its growth has been inhibited.

Some drugs which are used for urinary tract infections inhibit the growth of bacteria in the bladder until they are eliminated during urination.

Drugs that kill bacteria are bactericidal. These drugs are particularly useful in situations in which the normal host defenses cannot be relied on to remove or destroy pathogens.

A given drug can be bacteriostatic in one situation and be bactericidal in another situation, depending on the concentration of the drugs and the growth stage of the microorganism. Amoxicillin is a strong bactericidal drug which kills bacteria cells permanently.

Spectrum of the Activities of Amoxicillin

Antimicrobial drugs vary with respect to the range of microorganisms they kill or inhibit. Some kill or inhibit a narrow range of microorganism, such as Gram-positive bacteria, while others affect a wide range, generally including both Gram-positive and Gram-negative organisms.

Antimicrobial that affects a wide range of bacteria are called *broad-spectrum* antimicrobial. Examples are Amoxicillin and penicillin.

These are very important in the treatment of acute life-threatening diseases when immediate antimicrobial therapy is needed and there is no time to culture and identify the disease-causing agent.

The disadvantage of broad-spectrum antimicrobial therapy is that, by affecting a wide-range of organisms, they disrupt the normal flora that plays an important role in excluding pathogens.

Antimicrobials that affect a limited range of bacteria are called *narrow-spectrum* antimicrobials. Their use requires identification of the pathogen, but they cause less disruption to the normal flora.

Possible Effects of Combination of Amoxicillin with other Antimicrobials

Combinations of antimicrobials are sometimes used to treat infections, but care must be taken when selecting the combination because some drugs will counteract the effects of others.

When the action of one drug enhances the activity of another, the combination is called *synergistic*. In contrast, combinations in which the activity of one interferes with the other are called *antagonistic*. Combinations that are neither synergistic nor antagonistic are called *additive*.

How Amoxicillin Suppresses the Normal Flora

The normal flora plays an important role in host defense by excluding pathogens. When the composition of the normal flora is altered, this happens when a person takes an antimicrobial drug, pathogens normally unable to compete might multiply to high numbers.

Individuals who take broad-spectrum antibiotics orally sometimes develop the life-threatening disease called *antibiotic-associated colitis,* caused by the growth of toxin-producing strains of *Clostridium difficile.*

This organism is not usually able to establish itself in the intestine due to competition from other bacteria. When the normal intestinal flora are inhibited or killed, however, *Clostridium difficile* can sometimes flourish and cause disease.

Toxic Effects of Amoxicillin

Several antimicrobials are toxic at high concentrations or occasionally cause adverse reactions. For example, aminoglycosides can damage kidneys, impair the sense of balance, and even cause irreversible deafness.

Individuals taking these drugs must be closely monitored because of the very low therapeutic index. Some antimicrobial have such severe potential side effects that they are reserved for only life-threatening condition.

𝒞hapter Three

Diseases that can be treated with Amoxicillin

Amoxicillin is used for the treatment of the following diseases:

- Acute and chronic bronchitis.
- Typhoid and paratyphoid fever.
- Prosthetic joint infections.
- Helicobacter pylori eradication.
- Acute bacterial sinusitis.
- Lyme disease
- Acute otitis media (middle ear inflammation).
- Acute streptococcal pharyngitis and tonsillitis.

- Community-acquired pneumonia.

- Acute cystitis (inflammation of the bladder).

- Asymptomatic bacterial infection in pregnancy.

- Acute pyelonephritis.

- Dental abscess with spreading cellulitis.

Acute and Chronic Bronchitis

Acute Bronchitis

One of the most common ailments, especially among children and frail adults, is acute bronchitis. In most people myriads of germs lurk in the nose and throat, ready to find their way into the air passages and cause trouble there.

In many cases acute bronchitis develops as a complication of the common cold. In children, enlarged adenoids and diseased tonsils may have much to do with the tendency to repeated attacks of acute bronchitis.

In some adults, there appears to be a peculiar lack of resistance to this condition. In others, allergy plays an important causative role.

Exposure to cold from improper clothing may be conducive to bronchitis. Along with the chilling there is a lowering of resistance, and the alert germs take advantage of the opportunity to break through the protective tissues.

Bronchitis is a common complication of measles, scarlet fever, whooping cough, influenza, typhoid fever, and other infections. Chlorine and some other gases or fumes accidentally encountered in chemical laboratories or manufacturing establishments can produce severe forms of acute bronchitis.

The early symptoms of a typical case of acute bronchitis are; mild fever, mild headache, chilliness, some hoarseness and wheezing, a persistent but at first unproductive cough, and a sensation behind the breastbone.

When the cough becomes productive, the feeling of distress behind the breastbone usually lessens or subsides. Ordinarily, acute bronchitis runs its course in a few days, but it may become persistent, lingering on for months and finally becoming chronic bronchitis.

Chronic Bronchitis

Chronic bronchitis may develop after one or more attacks of acute bronchitis, but many cases that are thought to be chronic bronchitis may be something more serious, such as pulmonary emphysema, tuberculosis, or bronchiogenic carcinoma in adults. It may complicate or follow any disease or condition which involves protracted or repeated irritation or inflammation of the lining of the bronchial tubes.

In the 1964 report of the US Surgeon General's Advisory Committee, which had been given the assignment of studying the relationship between smoking and health, it was stated that cigarette smoking is the most important of the causes of chronic bronchitis in the US and increases the risk of dying from chronic bronchitis.

A dry cough, worse in the mornings, is characteristic. The cough is more severe and more likely to bring up sputum in the wintertime and following a cold. Wheezing and difficulty of breathing eventually develop in many cases.

Fever is rare. The condition may become worse from year to year, but since the discovery of antibiotics it has proved possible to bring about improvement in many cases of chronic bronchitis in which secondary bacterial infection is a factor.

Typhoid and Paratyphoid Fever

A specific germ, the typhoid bacillus, causes this acute, generalized, infectious disease. The body's lymphatic tissues are primarily affected. Symptoms include fever, a relatively slow heart rate, and, commonly, a rose-colored skin eruption. There is usually an enlargement of the spleen.

The germs of this disease are taken into the body through food or drink contaminated by bowel or kidney discharge from a typhoid fever patient or a carrier. One agent by which the germs are transferred to food is the common housefly.

The symptoms begin one to four weeks after the germs enter the body. The onset is usually gradual with a tire feeling and general weakness. There may be headache and nosebleed.

The fever rises higher each day until by the end of the first week it may reach 40 degree C higher in the evening than in the morning. The appetite is poor, the tongue is coated, and the teeth and lips are covered with a brownish deposit.

Diarrhea is common, especially at first, but there may be constipation instead. The stools have a very offensive odor. The abdomen is distended and tender to pressure.

After seven to ten days, small, rose-colored spots may appear on the skin, most abundant over the abdomen but sometimes on the chest and back also.

Near the beginning of the third week of illness, the fever usually begins to fall gradually. During the early part of the disease the face is flushed and the eyes are bright but by the second week the expression becomes listless and dull.

Cough is fairly common, especially early. As a rule, the skin is dry but sweating may occur late in the course of the disease, probably being the result of weakness.

The symptoms and the severity of typhoid fever vary greatly. The onset may be with convulsions, severe headache and delirium.

Many serious complications may develop, the most common being intestinal hemorrhage and intestinal perforation. When these occur, they usually come during the third week of the illness. The occurrence of intestinal hemorrhage is indicated by a sudden drop in temperature, a weak and rapid pulse, and a dark discharge from the bowel.

Intestinal perforation is indicated by sudden pain in the abdomen; mostly at the right side, a rapid drop in temperature, a spread of the abdominal pain to include the entire abdomen, and a weak but rapid pulse.

In some case of typhoid fever the symptoms are so mild that the patient feels it unnecessary for him to go to bed or to consult a Physician. Even in the mild cases, however, there is danger of intestinal hemorrhage.

It is the mild cases that create the greatest danger of transmitting the infection to susceptible persons, the reason being that the mildly ill person may be careless about the bowel and bladder.

Persons in reasonably good heath but whose bodies still harbor the typhoid bacillus to the extent that it is present in their bowel or bladder discharges are called "carriers".

A person who has a very mild attack of typhoid fever is just as likely to become a carrier as one who has a severe attack. It is in the effort to eliminate the carriers of this disease that the public-health departments insist on laboratory tests being made after a person recovers from this disease.

If the germs are still present in the body discharges, a course of treatment with the proper antibiotic drugs will usually remedy the situation.

One of the reasons that food handlers are required to have periodic examinations is to detect typhoid carriers. Many cases of the disease are traceable to food inadvertently contaminated by food handlers who are carriers of this infection.

In communities with poor sanitation, water is the most frequent means of transmitting typhoid fever. Food, especially milk, is the next most frequent offender. In urban areas, it is food that has been contaminated by healthy typhoid carriers that poses the greatest danger.

Paratyphoid fever: There are two varieties of paratyphoid fever, caused by germs much like those that cause typhoid fever: Paratyphoid A and Paratyphoid B.

Fever of either type tends to run a shorter course and tends to be less severe than typhoid fever, but the patient should receive similar care, and the same precautions should be taken against the spread of infection to other people.

Helicobacter pylori (Peptic/Stomach Ulcer)

Peptic ulcers are quite common. A peptic ulcer can either be in the stomach or in the duodenum, but only in regions exposed to the action of the acid and pepsin of the gastric juice.

Depending on their location, peptic ulcers are also called either gastric ulcers or duodenal ulcers. The ulcer victim often believes he has only indigestion or heartburn. On the other hand, typical ulcer symptoms may be only functional due to nervous tension, with no true ulcer present.

Peptic ulcer seems to be produced by the gastric juice's digesting away a small area of the gastric of duodenal mucous membrane that has been injured in some way or that has had its nutrition impaired by interruption of the blood supply to that particular area.

Gastric juice is normally present in the stomach, and it enters the duodenum along with partially digested food. Peptic ulcer is commonly found in people who have hyperacidity, yet some ulcer victims have normal or even low acidity.

It is a well-established fact that overwork and mental or emotional strain tend to cause or prolong peptic ulcers. So does the use of coffee and alcohol.

It is thought that these condition and habit may act through the autonomic nerves to have a constricting effect on the small arteries serving the lining tissues, thus reducing the resistance to acid and permitting a peptic ulcer to develop.

With peptic ulcer, there is usually pain and a definite point or small area of tenderness in the upper part of the abdomen. The pain is burning or boring in character, as a rule, and is most noticeable when the stomach is empty. It is often relieved by eating something, especially oily foods, but it tends to return as soon as digestion is well under way, or at least by the time the stomach or duodenum is again empty. It may also be relieved by taking an alkali, such as baking soda.

In severe cases, the ulcer may eat into the blood vessel and cause hemorrhage, perhaps slight and detectable only on chemical examination of the stools or it may be severe, causing the vomiting of large amounts of blood, accompanied by or followed by black, tarry stools. Neglected cases may even prove fatal.

Loss of weight is often a prominent symptom in persistent ulcer cases. The patient is sometimes afraid to eat. On the hand, gain in weight may be rapid when the proper treatment is begun.

There is significant difference in the probability of cancer in the two types of peptic ulcer. Duodenal ulcers are almost never malignant but gastric ulcers are commonly so.

A gastric ulcer that persists longer than three weeks should receive thorough scrutiny and appropriate surgical treatment, if indicated, because of high risk of its being malignant.

Perforation of the stomach or duodenal wall at the site of an ulcer may occur. It comes on suddenly, with a severe stab of pain in the abdomen, profound shock, rapid pulse, rising temperature, and sometimes a chill.

The abdomen becomes tender and rigid. Without prompt surgery, peritonitis sets in and is likely to prove fatal. Occasionally, however, the perforation develops so gradually that the escaping gastric or duodenal contents are walled in the symptoms are so mild that the condition may not be recognized for what it really is.

While life may not be in danger in such case, adhesions form and may make trouble later. All during the course of a peptic ulcer, therefore, careful watch should be kept to detect any symptoms of perforation, so that surgical repair will not be neglected.

Acute Bacterial Sinusitis

Certain cavities in the bones of the face and the floor of the skull are called sinuses. These cavities are lined with mucous membrane. All of them have openings communicating directly or indirectly with the nasal passages, and whenever an excess of mucous is secreted it must drain out through these openings into the nose or else build up pressure and create discomfort inside the sinuses.

Such congestion often builds up in case of allergy or a common cold. If there is no infection present, the trouble may correct itself soon but if pus-producing germs begin to work in the clogged sinuses, inflammation results.

The maxillary sinus is located in the cheekbone below the eye; the frontal sinus, in the frontal bone above each eye. Several small ethmoid sinuses are located in the ethmoid bone between the nasal cavities and the orbits if the eyes.

The sphenoid sinus or group of sinuses is situated in the sphenoid bone at the base of the skull, deep behind the ethmoid cells. The ethmoid sinuses become infected easily, but they also drain easily, so they may be responsible for a more or less persistent discharge but rarely cause acute sinusitis.

The maxillary sinuses also become infected easily, but they do not drain as readily as do the ethmoid sinuses. Acute maxillary sinusitis is, therefore, fairly common and it also often progresses to chronic sinusitis with a slow but persistent discharge, which tends to dry into crusts inside the nasal passages.

Frontal sinusitis is rather rare, but the drainage passages from these sinuses are long and narrow, so they easily become obstructed. As a consequence, frontal sinusitis is usually acute and painful and may require surgery for relief. Sphenoid sinusitis is very rare.

In general, acute sinusitis causes tenderness in the affected area, usually considerable pain, and a moderate fever.

Chronic sinusitis may produce few or no local symptoms, but if there is no free drainage for the pus, toxic substances may be absorbed into the circulation, impairing general resistance to diseases.

It is difficult and often impossible to apply any local treatment that will reach the germs inside the sinuses and clear up the infection. Suitable antibiotics such as amoxicillin taken by mouth or by injection are often beneficial especially in acute cases. These of course, must be ordered by your doctor.

Acute Otitis Media (Middle Ear Inflammation)

Inflammation of the middle ear is usually caused by germs that have spread from the nose or throat through the auditory tube to the ear. As a rule, it is a common cold that gets the germs started on this path.

The infection may be forced into the ear by pressure in the nose and throat when the nose is blown. It is a bad habit to blow the nose forcibly.

Middle ear infection also occurs as a complication in attack of scarlet fever, influenza, measles, or other diseases in which the throat becomes inflamed. The attack begins with pain in the ear. The pain may spread over the side of the head.

The victim may have chills and fever. The ear feels full. There may be ringing in the ear and partial or complete deafness. When the drum ruptures and lets the pus escape, there is prompt relief from pain, but a persistent discharge of pus begins.

Babies often have middle ear infection. When babies have this trouble, they cry constantly, turning his head from side to side and, unless they are too young to do so, placing their hand frequently upon the affected ear. Most times they have convulsions and fever as well.

Two great dangers attend middle-ear infection. First, the infection may spread to the mastoid cells behind the ear, and from them to the covering of the brain or to the blood vessels of the brain, causing death from meningitis or from thrombosis of these vessels.

Secondly, if the drum ruptures by itself, the ragged hole thus caused does not heal easily and may result in damage to the hearing. Professional advice and treatment are very important. The infection should be checked as soon as possible to keep it from spreading and the physician may have to make an incision in the eardrum to prevent spontaneous rupture and to facilitate aftercare.

Some cases of inflammation of the middle ear are not caused by infection but by congestion in the air passages or by obstruction of the auditory tube.

They may not cause fever or any severe pain, but there is often a sense of pressure or a snapping or ringing in the ears and an impairment of hearing.

These cases, as well as the aftercare of many others that started as infections, often require special treatments that must be given by a physician experienced in handling ear diseases, if the victims are to be relieved of their distressing symptoms and to have their hearing saved from permanent impairment.

Acute Streptococcal Pharyngitis and Tonsillitis

Acute streptococcal pharyngitis is also known as septic sore throat. This severe sore throat is caused by a strain of hemolytic streptococcus very similar to that which causes scarlet fever. In fact, there is very little difference between streptococcal sore throat and scarlet fever as far as the disease processes are concerned, there being in both a serious infection in the tissues of the pharynx.

But in scarlet fever there is in addition a skin rash caused by the effect of the toxin on the capillaries of the skin. Streptococcal sore throat occurs both as isolated cases and in epidemic form. Epidemics of this disease are usually the result of a streptococcal contamination of milk or milk products.

Spread of the disease from person to person is usually by contamination of articles of food and drink by germs derived from the throat of someone ill with the disease.

The potent toxin produced in the infected tissues of the pharynx makes the patient very weak. The possible complications of streptococcal sore throat include arthritis, persistent infection of the lymph nodes in the neck, middle-ear infection, occasional infection of the lining of the heart, and damage of the delicate tissues of the kidneys.

Antibiotic drugs are very effective against such infection. Amoxicillin is a good example of such antibiotic drug that could be used.

Acute Tonsillitis, on the other hand is a common disease among young people, many of whom have repeated attacks. This condition may be associated with rheumatic fever. It may be followed by infection of the heart valves, by red and boggy swellings under the skin or by acute inflammation of the kidneys.

These complications may also develop in connection with a tonsil infection that persists and becomes chronic, though no longer causing symptoms characteristic of acute tonsillitis. For this reasons, either children or adults who suffer from repeated attacks of acute tonsillar infection without acute symptoms should have their tonsils removed. This is done, of course, after the infection has subsided.

In acute tonsillitis the onset is often accompanied by a chill and aching in the back limbs. There is intense soreness of the throat, with great difficulty in swallowing.

The tongue is coated, and breath is foul. The tonsils are swollen and red, and they may show yellowish or whitish patches on the surface.

The neck glands are usually swollen. In some cases the entire throat is bright red, and there may be a red rash over the chest or the entire body. In such cases the infection is due to germs the same as, or similar to, those which cause scarlet fever.

Community-acquired Pneumonia

Pneumonia is a disease of the lungs in which the delicate lung tissue becomes acutely infected. Several kinds of germs and viruses may cause such an infection.

When the infection involves principally a certain lobe of a lung, the disease may be called lobar pneumonia. When the infection is scattered throughout the lungs and involves the delicate tissue closely related to the bronchi, it may be called bronchopneumonia.

There are two different reasons why pneumonia is a serious disease:

1. The toxemia is usually relatively great.
2. One's very life depends on the continuous function of the lungs.

In diseases of the digestive systems a person may go without food for s while, thus giving the affected organs to rest from their usual functions during the process of healing. But the lungs must function continuously day and night, whether they are involved with disease or not, in order that oxygen and carbon dioxide might be exchanged to satisfy the needs of the cells of the body.

If their involvement with disease curtails their function too much, death may result. Prior to the advent of antibiotic drugs, pneumonia in its various forms was one of the major killers.

Now the picture is markedly changed. Pneumonia, untreated, is still a serious, even fatal, disease. But with the early and proper use of antibiotic drugs, most of the types of germs which cause pneumonia can be rendered harmless even while the tissue resistance to the germs is being developed.

The germs and viruses which cause the various forms of pneumonia are widely prevalent, and almost everyone is exposed to them repeatedly.

Pneumonia Caused by Pneumococcus

In inflammation of the lung caused by pneumococcus germ there is a sudden onset of illness with violent chills accompanied by a rapidly mounting fever up to 40.6 degree C, chest pain on breathing, cough, and the spitting of rust-colored sputum.

The breathing becomes rapid with respiration up to forty per minute. When untreated pneumococcus pneumonia runs its course in about two weeks, ending in death in more than 30 percent of cases and in prompt improvement in the remaining 70 percent.

Common complications are pleurisy, empyema, lung abscess, infection of the heart and meningitis. In cases treated with antibiotics, the mortality rate is less than 5 percent.

Pneumonia caused by other Bacteria

Recently, an increasing proportion of pneumonias are caused by a single bacterial organism other than the pneumococcus. These include streptococcus, staphylococcus and bacillus.

The illness in these cases may have either a sudden or gradual onset. It usually develops secondary to some other illness such as a virus infection, viral pneumonia, influenza, measles, or some disease. Common complications in these cases include pleurisy, empyema and lung abscess.

Acute Cystitis (Inflammation of the Bladder)

In women, inflammation of the bladder often develops a day or two after sexual intercourse. In such cases, the bacteria that cause the inflammation have travelled up the urethra to the bladder. Inflammation can also occur as a complication of infection of the kidney.

In men, it may accompany infection of the kidney or it may follow an inflammation of the prostate. Any partial obstruction to the outflow of urine so that a residual amount of urine remains in the bladder at all times, favors the development of infection within the bladder.

The symptoms relate mostly to the functions of the bladder and include burning on urination, a desire to void frequently, and a feeling of urgency to empty the bladder at once.

General symptoms such as fever are usually caused by inflammations of other organs (kidney or prostate) rather than by inflammation of the bladder itself.

The usual case of inflammation of the bladder responds readily to appropriate treatment. If the aggravating cause is an obstruction to the outflow of urine, as an enlarged prostate or a stricture of the urethra, such condition must be corrected.

If the condition subsides and recurs repeatedly, there is some underlying cause which should be discovered and corrected.

Acute Pyelonephritis

The pelvis of the kidney is the enlarged upper end of the ureter, which is the tube that conveys the urine from the kidney to the bladder. Pyelitis, or inflammation of the kidney pelvis, may be caused by pus-producing bacteria.

These bacteria may arrive through the bloodstream flowing through the kidney, or they may come upward through the ureter from an infected bladder.

If the kidney substance is also involved, which is usually the case, the condition should be called pyelonephritis. Infected tonsils, infected teeth, or other foci of infection are sometimes apparently the original source of the bacteria.

One of the most common and persistent of the bacteria causing Pyelitis or pyelonephritis is the colon bacillus, which always abounds in the large intestine.

If not cleared out by thorough treatment, colon bacilli may remain in the pelvis of the kidney for years. These bacilli are often very resistant to treatment, and after apparent recovery recurrence of the infection is common.

A tendency to frequent voiding of urine may be the only symptoms with mild infections. At other times the inflammation is so great that there is a constant painful desire to void.

There may be severe chills, high fever, headache, nausea, vomiting, and extreme prostration for days at a time. There may be tenderness over the kidney region in the back. The distress, however, is often apparently confined to the bladder.

In fact, many people have had bladder treatments for a long time, when the real trouble was in the kidneys. If

Pyelitis becomes chronic, destruction or degradation of the kidney tissue may progress until it becomes so extensive that surgical removal of the kidney is the only way to cure the disease.

For this reason it is important to determine as early as possible whether one or both kidneys are involved and how far the infection has progressed.

Apparently, if both kidneys are infected, the removal of either one cannot be considered, and suitable treatment must be started early enough to make surgical removal of a kidney unnecessary.

Pyelitis seldom proves fatal unless neglected, but a cure often requires expert and persistent treatment. In some cases the most effective treatment a specialist can give is dilation of the ureters so the kidneys can drain away the urine more easily.

ᦞ *Chapter Four* ᦞ

Amoxicillin Adverse Reactions

The following are potential adverse effects that might happen as a result of overdosing, taking Amoxicillin with the incorrect drugs, experiencing drug interactions, or taking the medication at the incorrect time:

- Black Stool.
- Yellow skin and eyes.
- Safety warning, wheezing, unusual bleeding or bruises.
- Chest pain.
- Flushing and coughing.

49

- Back Rash.

- Stomach or abdominal pain or discomfort.

- Distension and blood in the urine (Hematuria).

- Bloody Nose.

- Headache.

- Stomach and leg pain.

- Generalized Body Swelling.

- Identify red patches on the skin.

- Eyelid puffiness or swelling around the eyes, lips, tongue, or face.

- Trouble Swallowing.

- Fast Heartbeat.

- Lightheadedness.

- Brittleness and Peeling.

- Gums that Bleed.

- The Skin Loosening.

- Urine that is dark.

- Diarrhea,

- Trouble Breathing, and Fever.

- Sore Throat.

- Urinary Tract Pain.

- Light Skin.

- Red and Angry Eyes.

- A tooth's discoloration.

- Feeling Uncomfortable.

- Heavy menstrual cycles.

- Welts.

- Joint and muscle pain.

- Appetite loss, aches in the muscles.

- Blisters, or Welting.

- A Quickly Decreasing Urine Amount.

- Swelling Lymph Nodes.

- Tenderness.

- Increased Thirst.

- Joint Inflammation.

- Itching and Redness.

- Skin that is sore and itchy.

- Ulcers or Sores.

- White Spots on the Lips and Mouth.

- Sores.

- Tightness in the Chest.

- Vomiting.

- Dislikable Breath Odor.

- Agitation.

- Weird Behavior and Confusion.

- Convulsions.

- Lower back pain and other pain.

- Sleeplessness.

- White Spots on the Tongue and Lips.

- Losing Weight.

- Vomiting Blood.

- Bloody or watery diarrhea.

- Breathe Shortness.

- Unusual weakness or fatigue.

- Poor, Odd, and Disappointing Taste, Taste Change.

Some of the aforementioned negative effects may infrequently not occur when using this medicine, while others may. Some side effects, however, might not require medical treatment since they might go away on their own without the need for a medicine to provide quick relief.

In conclusion, after using Amoxicillin prescription, do not hesitate to contact your personal doctor if you have any persistent adverse effect signs or symptoms within 48 hours.

Amoxicillin Interactions with Drugs

When Amoxicillin medication is used in combination with other drugs to treat certain chronic bacterial infections, chemical reactions in the body systems of consumers can result in mild to severe allergic reactions, including the side effects listed above, which can be fatal if the persons do not seek immediate medical attention to stop the escalation of the side effects in the body system.

You should thus be aware of the typical drugs that might lead to Amoxicillin drug indications. The drugs listed below are:

- Chloramphenicol.

- Tetracyclines,

- Sulfonamides,

- Clarithromycin,

- Rifabutin,

- Cotraceptive Pills For Birth Control.

- Erythromycin.

- Probenecid.

- Methotrexate.

- Allopurinol.

➢ Rifampin,

➢ Azithromycin.

Amoxicillin Effects In Pregnant And Nursing Women

Fertility in women and pregnancy

Amoxicillin is a great medication to use during nursing and throughout pregnancy. It efficiently stops bacterial infections from harming fetuses or unborn children and has no negative effects on a woman's ability to conceive.

Little child or newborn

However, there is no evidence to support the claim that Amoxicillin interferes with the mammary gland's ability to produce milk for a newborn to ingest. However, it is advised against breastfeeding your child while you are taking Amoxicillin since any unintentional chemical interaction with breast milk might pose a serious health risk to your child.

Hence, a nursing woman who is taking Amoxicillin is expected to tell her personal doctor before she breastfeeds her new baby. Before beginning to use Amoxicillin, a lactating mother should obtain a qualified doctor's approval and fully disclose her medical history to ensure proper supervision and appropriate prescription.

Amoxicillin Safety Warnings

Before you start using Amoxicillin medication, let your doctor know.

Amoxicillin medication reduces the effectiveness of vaccination. As a result, avoid using Amoxicillin while receiving immunizations.

To avoid an interaction with Amoxicillin, you must get your doctor's approval before combining any medications.

Openly discuss your medical details with your qualified doctor, who is able to determine whether your wellbeing can withstand the chemical reaction of amoxicillin without experiencing any negative side effects, regarding important organs like the liver or kidney malfunctions and viral infections.

If you are not told to use amoxicillin during pregnancy or nursing, strictly abide by your doctor's instructions when using amoxicillin medication.

The risk of Amoxicillin medication becoming deposited in breast milk might jeopardize the health of the child who ingests it. To get the best medical advice for you and your new baby, see your personal doctor.

How Amoxicillin is Helped by Augmentin

The antibiotic Augmentin includes a penicillin type ingredient that makes it active and more sensitive to a number of bacterial infections that can lead to chronic disorders. The pace of healing is accelerated when augmentin and amoxicillin are used together to treat bacterial infections.

Clavulanic acid, which is found in Augmentin medication together with Amoxicillin, increases the degree of bacterial infection cure and lowers the possibility of Amoxicillin medication adverse effects.

Therefore, Augmentin is regarded as a combination antibiotic that boosts therapeutic benefits in treating bacterial diseases including bronchitis, tonsillitis, sinusitis, pneumonia, and ear infections.

Augmentin is used to fight infections that can lead to bronchitis, gonorrhea, lung and skin infections, throat infections, and middle ear infections among other conditions.

Many difficult and serious bacterial illnesses and inflammation are frequently treated with the drug combination Augmentin and Amoxicillin.

When the defensive bacteria in the colon are completely eliminated by augmentin and amoxicillin, a particular bacterium like Clostridium difficile will grow and swiftly proliferate in the colon, causing inflammation.

Possible Negative Effects of taking Augmentin and Amoxicillin together

Due to the body's reactivity and the patient's tolerance to their therapeutic impact, Augmentin and Amoxicillin taken together can cause irregular side effects or moderate allergic reactions. As a result, your personal physician must provide thorough medical monitoring while you take both antibiotics because they are potent medications.

These are only a few of the frequent negative effects that some patients with poor body tolerance may experience when taking Augmentin and Amoxicillin. They include heartburn, rashes, itching, nausea, vomiting, bleeding, allergic reactions, and a host of other symptoms.

Chapter Five

Dosages of Amoxicillin for Various Illnesses

Amoxicillin medication comes in a variety of dosages that are designed to treat various bacterial infections in both children and adults.

Amoxicillin is the active component of therapeutic antibiotics designed for children, which come in dosages of 20 mg, 25 mg, and 30 mg respectively, while in dosages for adults of 150 mg, 200 mg, and 500 mg, respectively.

Different Amoxicillin manufacturing businesses offer the Amoxicillin dosage in varied strengths. According to the common bacterial diseases that may be treated right away, they manufactured Amoxicillin dosages, which in turn increased demand for Amoxicillin and the profitability of the businesses.

Before Amoxicillin is produced, a medical survey on the most common bacterial infections is crucial. This approach in eliminating bacterial endemic illnesses involved dose variation. You must inform your personal doctor about all of your medical history in order to receive a precise prescription for a specific healing dose of amoxicillin under close doctor's supervision, without you suffering any side effects during or following the use of amoxicillin medicine. This will ensure that amoxicillin is used correctly and has the best healing effect on both children and adults.

Precise Amoxicillin Formula for Children

Amoxicillin is manufactured in a liquid suspension or syrup to hasten dispersion and increase the effectiveness of the antibacterial action.

Adult Amoxicillin Formula

Amoxicillin is created to be compatible with the adult body's general systemic circulation and to enable effective delivery of Amoxicillin to the affected area. As a result, the medications amoxicillin and azithromycin are made as tablets, capsules, and injections. These are the most effective ways to treat different bacterial problems using amoxicillin medication.

Recommended Dosage for Adults and Children Greater than or Equals 40kg

Dosage for Acute bacterial sinusitis, acute pyelonephritis, dental abscess with spreading cellulitis, and acute cystitis

Take 250-500mg for every 8 hours or take 750mg for every 12 hours. If the infection is severe, take 750mg for every 8 hours.

Dosage for Acute otitis media, acute streptococcal tonsillitis and pharyngitis, and acute exacerbations of chronic bronchitis

Take 500mg every 8 hours or take 750 mg every 12 hours. For severe infections, take 750mg every 8 hours for about 10 days.

Dosage for Community-acquired pneumonia

Take 500mg of amoxicillin every 8 hours.

Dosage for Typhoid and Paratyphoid Fever

Take 500mg of amoxicillin every 8 hours.

Dosage for Prosthetic Joint Infections

Take 500mg of amoxicillin every 8 hours.

Dosage for Lyme Disease

For early stage, take 500mg every 8 hours up to a maximum of 4 g per day in divided doses for 14 days.

For late stage, take 500mg every 8 hours up to maximum of 6g per day in divided doses for 10-30 days.

Recommended Dosage of Amoxillin For Children Less than 40 Kg

Dosage for Acute bacterial sinusitis, acute otitis media, community-acquired pneumonia, acute cystitis, acute pyelonephritis, and dental abscess with spreading cellulitis

Take 20-90 mg per day in divided doses.

Dosage for Acute Streptococcal Tonsillitis and Pharyngitis

Take 40-90 mg per day in divided doses.

Dosage for Typhoid and Paratyphoid Fever

Take 100 mg per day in three divided doses.

Dosage for Lyme disease

For early stage, take 25-50 mg per day in three divided doses for 10-20 days.

For late stage, take 100 mg per day in three divided doses for 10-30 days.

Recommended Dosage for Children between 2-59 Months of Age with Pneumonia

Dosage for Fast-Breathing Pneumonia

For children between 2-12 months weighing 4 to less than 10Kg, give one tablet of amoxicillin dispersible tablet of 250 mg twice daily for 5 days.

For children between 12 months-5 years weighing 10-19kg give two tablet of amoxicillin dispersible tablet of 250 mg twice daily for 5 days.

Dosage for Fast-Breathing and Chest-Indrawing Pneumonia

For children between 2-12 months weighing 4 to less than 10Kg, give one tablet of amoxicillin dispersible tablet of 250 mg twice daily for 5 days.

For children between 12months-3 years weighing 10 to less than 14Kg, give two tablet of amoxicillin dispersible tablet of 250 mg twice daily for 5 days.

For children between 3-5 years weighing 14 to 19Kg, give three tablet of amoxicillin dispersible tablet of 250 mg twice daily for 5 days.

How Can I Make Up for a Missed Dose?

It is known as a missed dosage of amoxicillin if you truly neglected to take a preceding dose that you were intended to take at a specific time of the day. Make sure not to include the prior missed dose of Amoxicillin while taking the subsequent dose of the antibiotic.

If the time has passed two hours, do not worry using the missed dose; instead, wait for the next dose and use the exact dose for the period if the period interval is between six and eight hours and the previous missed dose was taken within the previous two hours when you remembered or had a chance to use it.

To prevent an overdose of Amoxicillin, which might be harmful to your health, do not combine the missed dosage with the preceding dose.

Warnings To Bear In Mind If You Take Too Much Of A Dose

Amoxicillin overdose suggests that you have taken an excessive amount. It is possible to overdose, but if you think you may have done so, call your doctor right away or the USA Poison Control Center at 1-800-222-1222 for immediate assistance.

This is done to avoid any potentially fatal bad effects that might exacerbate your medical issues and make the situation worse, endangering your life. The phone number is operationally available around-the-clock.

❧ *Chapter Six* ❧

Safe Online Pharmacy to Purchase Original Amoxicillin

Original Amoxicillin medication can be purchased with confidence from a reputable online pharmacy at a reduced price, in the neighborhood pharmacy, or as over-the-counter (OTC) medication close to your destination.

Additionally, you should be aware of the brand name that the manufacturer gives to Amoxicillin medications in order to avoid purchasing counterfeit versions of the drug.

This book will provide you the knowledge necessary to identify trustworthy online pharmacies that can provide you with real Amoxicillin at a discount. The medication amoxicillin may be repackaged in a refilling package with less than 21 pills or more. Although the refilled pills are noted on the packaging, the direct package also lists the brand name and the quantity of capsules or tablets within.

While other pharmaceutical firms use an acronym like Amoxil or the compound name Amoxihexol, Accord uses the name of the active component, Amoxicillin, as the brand name.

Amoxicillin is readily available from the online retailers and pharmacies listed below.

- HealthWarehouse: **www.healthwarehouse.com**

- WALGREEN: **https://www.walgreens.com/**

- EXPRESS-SCRIPTS: *www.express-scripts.com/*

- COSTCO WHOLESALE: **www.costco.com/**

- Dental-Directory: *www.dental-directory.co.uk*

- Pharmacy2U: ***www.pharmacy2u.co.uk.***

Dental Directory

Amoxicillin 500mg is cost-effectively priced.

All online pharmacies use the similar procedures, however individuals who don't have access to personal doctors or pharmacists are given additional care on the Pharmacy2u site.

Pharmacy2U

The location of Pharmacy2u is the United Kingdom (UK). If a consumer has a medical problem or needs further medical advice based on their medical history, the company has several medical professionals on staff, including doctors, pharmacists, and customer service personnel who are health-conscious.

You can take advantage of the free consultations and medical options indicated above.

How To Buy

- Type https://www.pharmacy2u.co.uk into the network tab of a web browser such as Google Chrome, Mozilla Firefox, UC Browser, Opera mini, etc.
- The homepage of Pharmacy2u will appear. Register with Pharmacology2U to create a new account by entering the personal data requested. You may receive greater discounts on each Amoxicillin medication you buy by opening an account.
- Type Amoxicillin Tablet into the search text box on the Pharmacy2U webpage and press the enter key on your laptop keyboard.
- The Amoxicillin 500mg Tablets detail page will display.
- Clicking on the amoxicillin container will bring up the amoxicillin website.

- Decide how much Amoxicillin you wish to purchase.
- Click "Check Out" to enter your shipping and payment details.

How to buy Amoxicillin on HealthWarehouse.com

- In the surfing network tab of Mozilla Firefox, Google Chrome, or UC browser, enter https://www.healthwarehouse.com.
- The homepage of HealthWarehouse.com will appear.
- Enter Amoxicillin Tablet into the search field using the computer keyboard or Tab Keypad. Amoxicillin 250 mg and 500 mg will be displayed right away.
- Select a 250 mg or 500 mg tablet container of Amoxicillin by clicking on it.
- Page presenting all available information on amoxicillin, including the quantity button, a picture of the medication, and the total amount due.

- Select the "Select" button next to the Amoxicillin pricing by clicking on it.
- Click the "Add to my Cart" button to bring up the Amoxicillin page.
- Choose the amount you like, then click "Check Out" to enter your shipping and payment details.

ॐ References ॐ

Brodie DP, Griggs JV, Cunningham K. Comparative study of cefuroxime axetil suspension and amoxicillin syrup in the treatment of acute otitis media in general practice. J Int Med Res 1990; 18(3): 235-239.

Calhoun KH, Hokanson JA. Multi center comparison of clarithromycin and amoxicillin in the treatment of acute maxillary sinusitis. Arch Fam Med 1993; 2(8): 837-840.

Sutherland R, Croydon EAP, Rolinson GN. Amoxicillin: a new semi-synthetic penicillin. British Med J 1972; 3: 13-16.

Eugene W. Nester, Denise G. Anderson, Evans C. Roberts, Nanacy N. Pearsall, Martha T. Nester.

Microbiology: A Human Perspective, Fourth Edition, 2004, 510-511.

Harold shryock, M.D. and Hubert O. Swartout, M.D, Dr.P.H. your health and you. The Stanborough Press Limited. 1980,Vol. 2 pg. 448-610.

Prankerd RJ. Critical compilation of pK , values for pharmaceutical substances. In: Harry G. Brittain, editor. Profiles of drug substances, excipients and related methodology: critical. 1st ed. Vol 33. London (UK): Academic press, an imprint of Elsevier; 2007.

Reeves DS, Bullock DW. The amino Penicillin: development and comparative properties. Infection 1979; 7 Suppl 5: 425-433.

Simar Preet Kaur, Rekha Rao, Sanju Nanda. Amoxicillin: A Broad Spectrum Antibiotic. International Journal of Pharmacy and Pharmaceutical Sciences. ISSN- 0975-1491. Vol 3, Issue 3, 2011, 30-37.

Subhas CM, Harsha R, Dinesha R, Thammanna GSS. Antibacterial activity of Coleus aromaticus leaves. Inter J of pharmacy and pharmaceutical sciences 2010; 2(3):63-66.

Torres RF, Consentino MO, Lopez MAB, Mochon MC. Simultaneous determination of 11 antibiotics and their main metabolites from four different groups by reversed-phase high-performance liquid chromatography–diode array–fluorescence (HPLC–DAD–FLD) in human urine samples. Talanta 2010; 81:871-880.

United States Pharmacopoeia-30 and National Formulary-25: The Official Compendia of Standards. Rockvile (US): United States Pharmacopoeial Convention; 2007. p.1402-1407.

Made in United States
Orlando, FL
08 December 2024

55236129R00046